I0416216

FINDING YOUR
INNER WARRIOR

A Guide for the Hesitant Woman
in the Wake of MeToo

FINDING YOUR INNER WARRIOR

A Guide for the Hesitant Woman in the Wake of MeToo

Nora Fahlberg

ELM HILL

A Division of
HarperCollins Christian Publishing

www.elmhillbooks.com

© 2019 Nora Fahlberg

Finding Your Inner Warrior

A Guide for the Hesitant Woman in the Wake of MeToo

All rights reserved. No portion of this book may be reproduced, stored in a retrieval system, or transmitted in any form or by any means—electronic, mechanical, photocopy, recording, scanning, or other—except for brief quotations in critical reviews or articles, without the prior written permission of the publisher.

Published in Nashville, Tennessee, by Elm Hill, an imprint of Thomas Nelson. Elm Hill and Thomas Nelson are registered trademarks of HarperCollins Christian Publishing, Inc.

Elm Hill titles may be purchased in bulk for educational, business, fund-raising, or sales promotional use. For information, please e-mail SpecialMarkets@ ThomasNelson.com.

Note: Some identifying details have been changed to protect the innocent from the guilty.

This book is presented solely for motivational and educational purposes. No warranties or guarantees are expressed or implied by author's choice to include any of the content in this volume, as results may vary. Neither the author nor the publisher shall be held liable or responsible to any person or entity with respect to any loss or incidental or consequential damages caused, or alleged to have been caused, directly or indirectly, by the information or program contained herein.

Library of Congress Cataloging-in-Publication Data

Library of Congress Control Number: 2019916891

ISBN 978-1-400329281 (Paperback)
ISBN 978-1-400329298 (Hardbound)
ISBN 978-1-400329304 (eBook)

Acknowledgments

I am so grateful for the people who have helped make this book happen. My transition from doormat to dauntless was long and slow, until three amazing people arrived in my life, one after the other.

The first is Ms. Janis Ware, an extraordinary entrepreneur and a wise, insightful person whom I'm honored to call a friend. She is one of those natural, warrior women—confident, assertive—everything I wanted to be. If every woman had a friend like Janis, the world would be a better place for both women and children.

Janis also introduced me to Dr. Viktor Bouquette, a brilliant, compassionate physician who also happens to be a magnificent warrior, trained in martial arts. His counsel was priceless. He took the assertiveness that I learned from Janis and grew my inner fighting spirit, so that I could tap into my warrior self when needed. Dr. Bouquette is another friend for whom I'll be eternally grateful.

The third is Reuben Goodgion, whom I dated for several years. He weathered the storm of my repressed anger, took Hagganah with me, and allowed me to beat on him (literally) as I learned to deal with emotions I had suppressed for so long. You can see Reuben taking a beating (and trying not to smile) in the photos in this book. Yet again, I'm so honored to have such a loyal, supportive friend.

Then, my new friends and creative team, Sean Waters, photographer and graphic wizard, and his partner, Sarah Birdsong, my website designer.

Without them and their considerable talent, support, and patience, I would have been lost when I took on this project.

My developmental editor, Krista Hill, helped me polish this work and guided me through the publishing process. I am so lucky to have found her. Last but not least, my brilliant husband, Gendo, whose generosity and support made this project possible.

TABLE OF CONTENTS

CHAPTER 1

ENOUGH IS ENOUGH

Once upon a time, I was a nice, quiet, sweet girl who tried to get along with everyone. As such, I had no idea what to do when, in my early teens, men began to harass and grope me. These incidents left me feeling grossed out, confused, and frustrated.

Hoping that men would eventually leave me alone or that someone would stand up for me didn't work very well. Actually, it didn't work at all. There weren't many options to change my predicament. I couldn't control men's behavior and I couldn't change the system. The only thing I *could* do was take charge of myself. Ultimately, I chose to recreate myself: to become more confident, more assertive—tougher.

It was a slow process that took far too long. Although I witnessed a few women calling out bad behavior here and there, I had no consistent role models. All of the girls and women I knew were passive like me. I read dozens of self-help books in an effort to discover the tools for my transformation. Little by little, over many years, I found the information I needed to start making changes. This guidebook contains all the things I wished someone had told me, or that I could have found in one source a long time ago.

The "consent movement" helped champion the idea that we shouldn't touch others without permission. As children, many of us were taught to keep our hands to ourselves; to me, this felt like we, as a society, were reinforcing this concept for those who didn't quite get the message. Then, #MeToo gave people an outlet to come forward and raise awareness about how prevalent harassment, assault, and rape are in our culture. Victims need forums for discussion and support, and more resources are now available.

Unfortunately, follow-up studies show that, for most women, not much has changed. Statistics say that approximately eighty percent of us have been harassed and that twenty-five percent of women will be assaulted in their lifetimes. I suspect it's higher than that. Many women told me stories that they had never reported. Some had never told anyone—not their husbands, boyfriends or family. And why would they? First, we know that we might not be believed. Then, we will likely be subjected to questions of what we did or didn't do that allowed the incident to happen.

During the summer of #MeToo, my friends shared their stories. One woman in her mid-twenties spoke of a job where one guy constantly grabbed and groped the female employees, using the common ploy of laughing it off as a joke. Another devout Christian southern lady in her seventies spoke of how, in her sixties, she had two separate incidents where men created excuses to reach down her shirt. Modest dress and age do not necessarily protect us.

Yet another woman had her booty slapped twice in once month: once by a stranger while she was bending over a dairy case at a store, and again by a friend of a guy she was dating. Her girlfriend asked her boyfriend when the woman could expect an apology from the friend. He replied that his friend had already apologized—to him. Not to the person he had assaulted, but to the man whose "property" he had violated! Upon hearing this, I was livid. I began sharing with her the strategies that would become this book.

Like many people who find their way into healthcare, especially fields of bodywork, I've always been the type of person in whom people felt they could confide. As a result, I heard stories of harassment and assault from friends, colleagues, and even strangers for years, beginning in high school. In addition to my own experiences, which I'll get to soon, I spent decades in healthcare, listening to hundreds of women's stories. I am a Chiropractic Physician, which might seem random and unrelated to this guidebook, except that it gave me the opportunity to be there for women who needed someone to hear them. When you put your hands on people to ease their pain, they often come to trust you with highly personal information.

As I worked on my patients, they would tell me everything. I listened, sympathized, and recommended counseling on a regular basis. However, due to negative perceptions of therapy, most of my patients insisted that they couldn't or wouldn't go to a psychologist, saying that they preferred to just tell me. So, I listened to horrific and heartbreaking stories as I worked to ease their physical aches and pains—and I kept their secrets, as I was and still am bound by doctor/patient confidentiality.

After two serious auto accidents just a few years apart, I had to retire early from full-time practice to heal my own body. I started teaching anatomy, physiology, and other healthcare sciences at a massage school and then at an acupuncture college, where my students told me their stories.

Next came the incidents related to me by the cast and crews in the film industry, where I worked part-time for over twenty years. On one project there was a serial offender, harassing and grabbing crew members regularly. He tried with me, but by then I was more assertive: I whispered in his ear that if he touched me, I'd break his fingers. He left me alone, but he was so relentless with the other women that I reported him on their behalf. But it didn't help.

The countless stories I heard had some common threads. Almost all the women felt guilt or a sense of shame. They wondered what they had done wrong, or what they shouldn't have done. They second-guessed normal, everyday choices that men never have to think about and beat themselves up with self-blame. They suppressed the anger they felt—or turned it against themselves.

We had another problem in common: we didn't know what to do

when it happened. Growing up, we all got the same programming, which definitely did not include standing up for ourselves. The most common response was freezing, followed by denial and self-blame. Most of us couldn't speak up for ourselves when men said suggestive, insulting, and vulgar things. And we had no idea what to do when they touched or grabbed us. Many of us were more concerned about making waves, or causing a scene, than the violation of our bodies.

It seemed like we had no control over if and when any random male would put his hands on us. After all, if we had done A, B, or C—or had not done X, Y, or Z—then it wouldn't have happened. We were "asking for it" somehow, or so certain men (and women) thought. "Boy will be boys" was the standard response.

A small percentage of men (and yes, sometimes women)—let's just call them "creeps"—have this idea that women, girls, *and* boys are theirs for the taking, that they are entitled to touch them whenever they want, and that society will defend them and give them cover—and it does. In a bizarre convolution of the concept "innocent until proven guilty", in cases of harassment and assault the victim is rarely presumed to be innocent. Can you imagine victims of a mugging, robbery, or arson being questioned about how they might have been "asking for it"?

Men started putting their hands on me when I was fifteen. When I was in chiropractic college, which was ninety percent male, I started asking the guys why they thought it happened so much. The feedback was that I was…wait for it…*too nice*. Lots of guys, they told me, see smiling and being friendly as a "green light". *Geez.*

Immediately, I started trying to project a colder, less friendly, less approachable persona. It was tough because I genuinely liked people—and men. But I figured it was worth a try. Also, during college I experienced a few intense, frightening incidents which I'll share in a bit. Those incidents woke me up and fueled my desire to change whatever I could to help me deal with future problems.

Fast forward to the summer of 2018, with #MeToo going strong. After my own experiences, reading people's stories, and hearing from young friends, I started to become angry—not for me, but for the younger generations who must deal with the same crap. I'd had enough of "Boys will be boys".

Something more, or different, needed to be done: something more proactive--and surely someone was doing something along the lines of what I had happened to figure out. But hours of research came up mostly empty for guidance in dealing with the incidents that occur in all areas of our lives.

Then, one morning at 3:00 am, I woke up and it hit me like a bolt of lightning: I had made it from doormat to defiant, so others could as well. I wrote a roadmap based on what had worked for me. My goal is to share it with the hope that it will help decrease the frequency and trauma of the incidents that girls and women—our friends, sisters, daughters, nieces, and granddaughters—might face as they go through life.

Recent social and political events have shown us the current state of women's and victims' rights, and it doesn't look good. We have always been blamed for being harassed, assaulted, and raped. Not only has it not gotten any better, but it appears to be getting worse. The "boys will be boys" mentality is on steroids, and the men in power have shown us that, yet again, we are not to be believed—if they even bother to listen.

Telling our stories doesn't protect us, and I'm not convinced that filing sexual harassment claims helps all that much, either. We get transferred, demoted, blacklisted, and fired. And harassment and assaults don't just occur in the workplace; they happen in stores and markets, at concerts and parties—with strangers and men whom we know, like, or even love.

Since our society is unable to protect us or give us justice, what can we do? I waited for years for others to help me and it didn't happen. Do you want to keep waiting for others to do the right thing, or have you had enough?

Alright. Let's take a minute to acknowledge how irritating it is that, yet again, change seems to be up to us. It's not fair. Yes, men should just behave. They should stop groping us. And stop raping. In a better world this might happen, but I've seen no sign of this world in my lifetime and now things seem to be moving backwards. I hate that this is the way things are. And yet, in my opinion, if there are a few more things that I can do that will help, that might make a difference, I'm going to do them. Even if my efforts don't always work, I can console myself knowing that I tried and free myself from any personal blame.

And if people are going to keep using the "boys will be boys" excuse—*and they are*—then maybe we need our own phrase. I'm going with "Women will be warriors." Why not? Your inner warrior can be in reserve and called upon whenever you need her. *But* you have to know how to connect with her…

CHAPTER 2

CONFESSIONS OF A
FORMER DOORMAT

My own stories begin with a normal, stable, happy childhood in the Midwest. My parents were strict, but not overly so, and religious in a moderate denomination. I was raised to be sweet and compliant, not to talk back or make a scene: it was a great recipe for becoming a doormat and a victim. While girls were trained to be "nice", boys got a free pass for poor behavior that lasted a lifetime—the "boys will be boys" excuse.

Although I was a tomboy with short hair who was often mistaken for a boy, as soon as I hit adolescence men began to grope me: not boys my age, but adults. When I grew longer hair and decided that I liked skirts and dresses, it got worse—adult men continued to help themselves to a feel or a squeeze. Some were men my parents knew and trusted, but many were strangers in public places. They were usually random, sneak attacks. I mostly froze, having no clue what to do (Freezing is a common response. We will come back to that later).

After several years of unwanted touching, the events that really woke me up were much scarier. One lovely summer day during college, while enjoying a bike ride, I was thrown from my bike when a guy slapped my booty from a moving car. I remember hearing "Hey baby!" before I felt the blow that sent me flying over the handlebars. The car sped off as I was in mid-air; luckily, I landed in a soft, grassy spot.

I lay on my back, looking up at a clear blue sky. As I checked my body for injuries, I heard a car door slam. Another car had stopped and someone came running up to me. He'd seen the whole thing and had stopped to see if I was ok, asking if I needed an ambulance.

Fortunately, I was mostly ok. I was shaken, with only minor scrapes and bruises, but I was angry. If that beautiful, soft grass had not been there, I could have been seriously injured—or worse. The jerk who hit me hadn't factored for the extra force that a moving vehicle would add to the slap: he could have killed me.

The next incident was the game-changer. It happened not long after the bike incident, on a girls' night out dancing at a nice, suburban club. My friends had gone for drinks, but I kept dancing. It was late in the evening, and the dance floor was full of people having a good time. Suddenly, I found myself surrounded by a group of about five guys. The memory of their polo shirts, khaki pants, and clean-cut looks is still fresh. I wondered why these guys were moving into my personal space. Suddenly, they had me trapped in the middle and began putting their hands all over me. Two hands were restraining my arms. They slipped their hands into my top and tried to put their hands down my pants. When they couldn't get my pants unzipped, they squeezed and grabbed whatever they could. It was a horrifying experience having all those hands grabbing my breasts, derrière, and crotch.

The attack had been coordinated, and I panicked for a moment as I realized that no one had noticed what was happening. No one was coming to save me. A surge of anger flowed through me and my instincts for self-preservation kicked in. I fought back, reflexively, and purely out of instinct because I had no training. I struck hard and fast, kicking a knee here and there, stomping on feet, biting a hand over my mouth hard enough to taste blood. When one let go of my right arm, I elbowed the guy immediately behind me. In just a few seconds, I had hurt most of them badly enough that they broke off the attack and headed straight for the door, leaving the club in a hurry like the cowards and bullies they were.

The rush of emotions that followed was intense. There was denial, as in "I can't believe what just happened", though I was still feeling the adrenaline. Mostly, I felt victorious—with a bit of righteous anger. People around me realized they had just witnessed a genuine fight, and that I had won. A couple of guys asked if I was ok. My friends returned from the bar and heard the tale of what they had missed.

The incident became known as the "group grope" among my friends, because one of my coping mechanisms is to poke fun at my bad luck. The story of this unusual bar fight got around my class, and I remember a few guys joked that they "wouldn't be messing with me". My girlfriends thought I'd feel traumatized, but I didn't. By fighting back, I no longer felt helpless. I had fought off multiple attackers by instinct alone: I could stand up for myself. I felt strong.

Unfortunately, I was a slow learner. I didn't yet have it in me to resist on a consistent basis, as I was still attached to the mindset and programming of being nice. I *needed* to be nice. What I didn't understand was that I could cultivate a fighting spirit and be nice at the same time.

In addition to physical attacks, I have lost or quit jobs due to harassment, had grades lowered by professors because I wouldn't sleep with them, and endured countless comments from both strangers and men whom I knew. I reported the professors at college and got nowhere—big surprise! At least I had spoken up.

When an ex-boyfriend assaulted and stalked me, I went to the police. At the time, there were no laws against stalking and the police told me the guy "just wanted me back". *Really?* Promising to kill me and choking me into unconsciousness were no big deal because he wanted me back? *Wow.*

I remember arguing with them, which was uncharacteristic of me, but I was petrified. Were they going to wait until he killed me to do anything? They insisted there was nothing they could do. They told me to buy a gun. On top of the trauma my ex had inflicted upon me, this felt like a punch in the gut. It was a wake-up call: I would have to protect myself.

Fortunately, my ex's family intervened and ended the immediate danger to myself. Still, my instinct for self-preservation had kicked in and I knew I would have to figure out how to fight back. I still had no idea that deep inside me was a warrior spirit.

About fifteen years later, my second and third stalkers occurred simultaneously (Did I mention that I have bad luck?). This pushed me over the edge and into my final breakthrough. Recalling the "group grope", it occurred to me that I could train myself to be ready to resist at any time. I could, and would, overcome my fears, my programming, and my habits and become a warrior.

Two close friends helped me to become more assertive. One taught me how to speak up, and what to say. The other began calling me "Boudicca"—after the Celtic queen who led armies against the Romans—to help me embrace my inner fighting spirit. I took eighteen months of a hard-core Israeli military self-defense system known as *Hagganah*. I allowed all the anger I had repressed for decades to flow through me, then channeled it as productively as I could. Anger can be functional if we don't allow it to blind us to our purpose.

The result was such that people who have only known me for the last twenty years can't believe that I was ever an easy target. I escaped the self-limiting conditions that made me passive. You can as well, if you are willing to do the work. The journey begins with re-evaluating the messages we absorbed while growing up, discarding the mindsets that no longer serve us, and cultivating our inner, fighting spirits.

CHAPTER 3

DISCLAIMERS

L et's establish some important disclaimers:

First, **even in those situations where we do not or cannot stand up for ourselves or fight back, it is still never, ever our fault.** It is always and forever the responsibility, blame, and shame of the creep. Sometimes, even when we are prepared, when we have the mindsets and have developed the reflexes to respond, there are circumstances where it might not help us.

It doesn't matter what we are wearing, if we are alone, if we have something or even too much to drink, or if we don't manage to fight back. None of this makes it our fault. Again, why is sexual harassment/assault the one crime where the victim is consistently presumed to have been part of the cause?

Second—not all men. Of course not. I adore men and have had lots of amazing guys as friends through the years. In fact, it was my male friends who encouraged me to fight back, verbally and physically, insisting that men in general and bullies in particular understand a show of force more than anything else. It is a minority of men (and sometimes women) who do these things, but they are often serial offenders.

Despite all my bad experiences, I think that most men are good guys and would try to help us if they could. I say this because most of the men

I've encountered, including acquaintances and strangers with whom I've crossed paths, could have harassed or assaulted me but did not. These men tend to be our allies, and there are more of them than there are creeps. To them, I say thank you. Thank you for being gentlemen. Please continue to be our allies!

Speaking of men, the solution that I propose—dealing with the incidents ourselves as they occur—is a lot more like how men handle conflict with each other. They have words, sometimes punch each other out, then go have a beer: it's over and they know where each other stands. Imagine what the average, heterosexual guy would do if another guy made a suggestive comment or smacked him on the rump. We can take a similar, straightforward approach, minus the punching because there are safer ways to fight back. This very example can help certain men "get it", if they dismiss harassment as no big deal. When they make sarcastic comments like, "I'd like to be harassed", they tend to assume it would be by someone to whom they are attracted.

It's been both sad and weird hearing guys describe incidents with the TSA as they join the ranks of MeToo. Men are assaulted as well and airport security has increased the frequency. One good friend described a prolonged fondling by a TSA agent, followed by denial and then self-blame, wondering if he had done something to provoke it. I listened and empathized before explaining to him that he had been sexually assaulted and it wasn't his fault. He was already an ally of women, and this made him even more so.

Some men, unfortunately, will never get it or will be creepy anyway. There will always be jerks, so I propose that we take a page from the men's playbook and learn to respond immediately and directly, with the show of strength they understand.

Third, I'm hoping to inspire women to transform themselves and find their inner warrior, and many are understandably irritated at being asked to do the changing. This is partly because the responsibility is always on us, and partly because the message that we "should" take responsibility has usually been packaged with the subversive message that if *we* haven't done enough, then it's our fault. I reject this subtext and I'm unhappy that it's come to this, so this is not the message I intend to share. My goal is to empower you so you'll have a better idea of how to take care of yourself.

Additionally, let's take back the word "victim", as it has somehow become an insult in and of itself. If you have been victimized, it does not take anything away from your self-worth. It doesn't have to mean that any facets of who you are have been damaged or stripped away. "Victim" simply describes an individual who has been wronged. Ultimately, in your own time and you own way, you can choose *not* to let that define you. Instead, you could see yourself as a survivor—which has become more mainstream—or, as a warrior who has done battle and taken a few hits, which is how I perceive myself. Ultimately, you have the power to choose how to define yourself.

CHAPTER 4

OVERCOMING THE CHALLENGES OF SAYING "NO"

A large part of the socialization of girls is training us to be passive and self-sacrificing. We are taught to put the needs, desires, and feelings of others first. Don't think of yourself or ask for anything back, as that makes you selfish. And don't say no—that isn't being agreeable. If you say no, then you have failed to be nice. Women are supposed to be the peacemakers, the ones who smooth over the rough patches, make others feel better, make boys and men feel manly and validated. So, when we tell them no, we are mean, cold, and heartless—not to mention all the other names we get called. And if someone touches you? From childhood, if a fellow student or neighbor boy pinched or hit me, they got the benefit of the doubt. They were just teasing or showing that they liked me. "Boys will be boys". If you think about it, this is a dangerous message to give to girls: if they hit you, it means they like you. No wonder women struggle with escaping domestic violence.

The messages that many women are repeatedly given throughout our formative years result in our having no idea how to speak up for ourselves. We usually aren't taught to fight back either, so we tend to freeze and become silent. Then, we suffer the unwarranted emotions of denial, guilt, and shame that usually follow an unwanted verbal or physical encounter.

On the other hand, I've encountered a few women who were natural warriors, who could easily stand up for themselves. Some couldn't understand why other women didn't just do the same, and I've tried to explain that they were lucky to have that ability. It is these women whom I have used as role models to re-train myself, and it is my hope that they will reach out and encourage more women to fight back. With these warrior role models in mind, the rest of us can create a new mindset for ourselves. This new mindset is focused on the idea that we are worthy of respect. We are worthy of countering rude comments, lewd requests, and criticism of our bodies. We are worthy of polite treatment, and especially of deciding who touches us and when. Our bodies are not public property.

With this idea, we will need to cultivate some new behaviors that will serve us well in all areas of our lives. We must learn to stand tall, speak our minds, and establish our boundaries. We can train ourselves to confidently say "No!", as well as take other measures if that doesn't get results. We can learn how to enforce our boundaries and call out incursions. And these are great skills to have, anyway.

We must also be ready for possible backlash. Be prepared for certain people to call us every name in the book, both perpetrators and their enablers. Name-calling is their way of reminding us of our supposed "place", forcing us to submit, to shut up, or to not be "overly sensitive".

But guess what? Having started out sweet, nice, and accommodating, I can tell you that I still got called names. So, since we're going to hear them regardless, let's hear them because we *resisted*. I believe that if we start this trend, changing our mindsets to confidence and resistance, it will get better not just for each of us individually, but for all of us.

Our current culture is unable or unwilling to call out and reprimand the creeps in the numbers needed to effect significant change. The status quo doesn't want change. The men who do these things don't want to be held responsible for their bad behavior. We can wish they would behave all we want, but they have more power than we do, so they don't have to.

And yet, we do have power. The men who do these things count on us to be passive and quiet. They count on being able to shame us into silence and submission. They count on being able to coerce us. When they can no longer count on any of that, because more and more women are fighting back, then, I believe, the tide will turn.

So, to get from doormat to dauntless, from silent to self-assured, from passive to powerful, we first change out mindsets and become more confident and assertive. To do this, we need to start at the beginning...

CHAPTER 5

Cultivating Self-Love/Esteem

Why am I starting here? Because as I listened to and tried to support the women who told me their stories, a common thread was that they had low self-esteem and couldn't imagine defending themselves because they didn't feel they were worthy. We all deserve to know, really know, in our hearts, that we are worthy of respect as a basic human right. So, we begin with the concept of self-esteem.

Old mindset: "I'm not good enough."
New mindset: "I am good enough."

I'm going to keep coming back to mindsets, because this is the key to change. The things that we tell ourselves about ourselves create our self-image. And our self-image dictates what we can and can't do.

How do we change our mindsets? Science! Specifically, using a trait of the brain called *neuroplasticity*, or brain plasticity. This is the ability of the brain to adapt, change, rewire, and be reprogrammed. Philosophers and sages have known for millennia that we can change not only our thoughts and our behaviors, but who we are. We now have the science to explain how it happens in the brain. It explains how things like repetition, chanting, meditation, prayer, hypnosis, and affirmations work. Neuroplasticity proves we can have more self-love and become more confident, even if we don't feel that way right now.

It saddens me to say, but after decades of listening to people (as men have confided in me as well), those of us with healthy self-esteem are rare. Most of us have low self-esteem. If you are among this majority and have poor self-esteem, if you don't love yourself, I know exactly how you feel. Decades ago, I felt that way, too. But I wanted to change, so I searched for a way out of the pain. In my case, it was Dr. Robert Schuller's book *Self Love*, which I can credit with preventing me from taking my own life around the age of nineteen.

For this project, I went looking for newer books and found one that I really liked by Kamal Ravikant, entitled *Love Yourself Like Your Life Depends On It*. It's a quick read with simple action steps. Kamal's first exercise is to counter the negative voice in your head with the phrase "I love myself". As you repeat this phrase over and over as a mantra to drive out negativity from your mind, you reprogram your brain. This book is worth its weight in gold. Please get yourself a copy.

When I shared this mantra with some friends, they protested that they couldn't tell themselves that they loved themselves. These were educated, professional women who couldn't express self-love. We kicked around some alternatives, so if "I love myself" is too much, start with something like, "I am learning to love myself" or "I love myself more every day" until you can finally say that you love yourself. And you deserve your love!

If these mantras trigger a backlash of negativity, which research suggests can happen with low self-esteem, it just means that you'll need to focus on becoming aware of and calling out the automatic thoughts that aren't allowing you to accept positive or loving thoughts about yourself. In the meantime, please don't give up on this, because you can still apply the rest of the ideas in this book while you build your self-esteem.

Research has indicated that self talk is the most critical element in improving our self-esteem. It is also called "internal dialogue", "automatic thoughts", etc., and when you pay close attention to these thoughts, you will notice that they tend to be negative. In his book *The Power of Now*,

Eckhart Tolle calls it the "Thinker", and describes how to manage it. A good friend of mine seems to have an extra-mean version, so we call his the "Stinker". Whatever we call it, most of us are constantly thinking the worst of ourselves and criticize ourselves non-stop. We bully ourselves, and this isn't healthy.

At this point, I'd like to note that negative thoughts are normal because they are part of our instincts to protect ourselves. Our ancestors who were more aware, more on guard, always watching for danger were more likely to survive. But when those thoughts become self-bullying, they have got to go. The path to changing them begins with monitoring your self-talk for these repetitive, negative thoughts and making a list so you can identify patterns. Next, evaluate them for what is true as opposed to something you've just accepted as true because you've been thinking it for so long. Call these thoughts out and question them. Begin to replace them with more positive versions. This process in diffusing negative and irrational thoughts is from a therapeutic approach called Cognitive Behavioral Therapy. Look it up online for more info, find a book about it, or if you can, see a psychologist who specializes in this therapy. It's really good stuff.

What if you can't see a psychologist for this? Well, then we are back to the books, and there are plenty of great books on this topic. There's also another alternative that we'll get to soon. In the meantime, as you start to monitor those negative thoughts, begin to think about their origin. Where did you get these ideas about yourself? When you do this, you'll probably realize that many of them go back to your childhood, or something unkind that someone said to you, and that you decided to accept them as true. Remember to question whether they really ARE true (Hint: They aren't).

Self-love/esteem can also be improved with creative visualization, guided meditation, and hypnosis, as they all use a similar approach of repetition. Any process that repeats the new message until you can truly accept it will work. I used to stick Post-it notes everywhere to remind me of my chosen mantras. While you figure out which combination of these methods of repetition best works for you, please remember that we have been taught to show respect, to be kind, sensitive, and caring toward others. Let's give ourselves some kindness, too. Learn to be your own best friend.

There are other things we can do to cultivate self-love and self-esteem. Countless books, magazine articles, and internet sources are available to help with this, but let's summarize some common tips here:

Self-awareness is also important for reducing negative influences. Think about what has impacted or continues to affect your self-esteem: family, or lack of family, friends, or lack of friends, peers, the media, body image, social media, etc. Once you figure out who or what makes you feel bad about yourself, avoid what you can. Excuse yourself and walk away, block the bullies, read something else. Ignore the negative.

Media is a huge offender, in my opinion. Studies have shown that girls and women feel worse about themselves after looking at women's magazines, because they are bombarded with pictures of "perfect" women. Not only do those women not look perfect in real life, they are very likely dealing with their own self esteem issues. And, they often represent a very narrow concept of beauty. We are all beautiful in our own, unique way.

Spend time with people who genuinely like/love you, people who lift you up. Limit the time you spend with people who leave you feeling drained or unhappy. Walk away from anyone who insults you, judges you, or otherwise diminishes you. You do not have to accept that kind of treatment.

If you are lonely, search out your tribe(s), preferably in real-life but online groups can help, too. Practice your listening skills. Ask people questions and you'll get conversation. Most people like to talk about themselves, so good listeners are often popular companions. Just make sure that you have someone to listen to you, too.

Focus on your positive qualities. We all have our strengths and weaknesses. Most of us get caught up in our weaknesses and downplay our strengths. Write a list of what you like about yourself. If you find this difficult, ask a friend or loved one to help.

I'll go one step further: I believe we all have a *superpower*. Figure out what your superpower is and cultivate it. Maybe it's that you bake amazing brownies or are good at gardening or organizing. We all have gifts: nurture yours.

Acknowledge and enjoy your successes. It doesn't matter if they are small, because big accomplishments are usually the result of small steps made up of a mixed bag of successes and failures. Only focus on your failures long enough to learn from them. Then, let them go.

Learn to accept compliments without making excuses. So many of us find ways to dismiss nice things that others say to us, when instead we could accept and remember those nice words when we are doubting ourselves.

Practice gratitude. Recent research has found that gratitude alters the heart and the molecular structure of the brain. It helps us detach from toxic emotions. Taking a few minutes every day to notice and reflect on what to be thankful for will increase your positive emotions, help you sleep better, and improve your immune system. Consider keeping a "gratitude journal" and try to express appreciation to the people in your life.

Find ways to challenge yourself. Find a hobby, join a class, or volunteer your time for something you feel passionate about. It doesn't have to be big—just do something. Start with small goals, like reading a book, drinking more water, or taking a daily walk—anything that can help you feel more positive about yourself.

Take care of yourself. Your health is important, so watch your stress levels, your food and drink choices, your exercise level, how much you sleep, etc. The information is out there, and you likely already know what would make you healthier. If you don't take care of yourself, who will?

Please reach out if you need help: get support if things become too much to manage. Get counseling if you can. Lots of organizations offer counseling at very low costs. If you can't do that, there are online services and 800 numbers to call. You are not alone.

There are lots of excellent books out there that can help. Find a few and read them. Although different authors may say essentially the same thing, you might have to search for the one that phrases it in a way that resonates with you. The repetition also helps with reprogramming your brain as you read.

And, there's good news! Even if you don't love yourself or have healthy self-esteem right now, you possess a natural instinct for self-preservation. This is your inner fighting spirit, your warrior self. So, in the meantime, we can work with that and begin to develop confidence.

CHAPTER 6

BUILDING AND PROJECTING CONFIDENCE

While you grow self-love and confidence, there are a few hacks you can do to "fake it until you make it". Again, most women have been socialized to be sweet, passive, and accommodating. We must now delete that programming, discard any old, unhelpful mindsets and replace them with something useful.

Old mindset: "I'm not good enough", "I can't do it", or "I'm a fraud."
New mindset: "I can do it" or, "I can learn and get better."

Anytime you catch yourself saying something negative to yourself, question it, then replace it with a more positive thought. Repeat as needed. Call out the thoughts that are holding you back.

Some meditation practices suggest labeling your thoughts and feelings to clarify, accept, and validate them. For example, when I, as an introvert, realized that I would need to make videos to post on the internet, I had quite a few negative thoughts run through my mind. So, I called them out. Doubt. Fear. Anxiety. Once I named the culprits, they were easier to overcome. *We all have these feelings.* The question is, do you let them stop you, or do you go on with your plans and your life despite them? I'd still rather not be on the internet, but this information is so important that I'm willing to move through my fears and anxiety to get it to you.

Practice the hacks I am about to list, so you will appear less vulnerable. As you use them, you will begin to feel more confident and begin retraining your brain. How? Science again! This time, the science of body language, or the unconscious and universal non-verbal messages we constantly send and receive. We are going to take this well-documented science and use it in our daily interactions to appear and feel more confident.

How do we apply it? First, we become aware of what we are currently communicating and then deliberately choose which non-verbal messages we send. There is a lot of research behind these suggestions, and if you can make even a few changes you will be perceived as being more confident, even if you aren't quite there yet. The more aware you become of your non-verbal communication, the more you practice projecting confident non-verbals, the faster your brain will use its plasticity to reprogram for true confidence. Here are some basics:

- Posture: Stand up straight. Shoulders back, arms down, head back and chin up. Compare how this looks and feels to rounded shoulders or slumping with the arms covering the body. The first communicates confidence, the second suggests insecure and vulnerable.

In one of the most viewed TED talks, "Your Body Language Shapes Who You Are", Dr. Amy Cuddy covers the non-verbals of posture. She focuses on how power-posing, specifically the pose she calls the "Wonder Woman" stance (heads up, shoulders back, feet apart, hands on hips) raises your confidence. She also updates "Fake it til you make it", to "Fake it until you become it". If you haven't seen this talk, I can't recommend it enough as it's brilliant.

- Gait: Walk with good posture and intent. This is especially important if you are in a vulnerable situation, as studies show that criminals can tell who will make an easy target in just a few seconds, based on posture and gait. Walk with your attention on your surroundings, notice who is around you, who is watching you, etc. And slow down a little. Moving quickly, as women often do, signals insecurity.

- Body orientation: Turning your torso and feet toward a person signals interest, so if someone is bothering you, keep your body turned slightly away from them.

- Eye contact: Looking away while speaking, especially in a downward, averted glance, is subconsciously interpreted as a sign of weakness and submission. Instead, look directly into someone's eyes when you speak. If this is hard to do, try looking at a point between their eyes, which can be somewhat unnerving for them.

- Gestures: Try to avoid touching your face, hair, or body around men whom you aren't interested in getting to know better, as this is read as flirting. You may just be nervous or distracted, but they unconsciously receive a message of interest, so it's important to be aware of it and stop it.

- Sound: When responding to something inappropriate, try to speak in a deeper or stronger tone than usual. Not necessarily loud, as sometimes lowering the volume and speaking sternly is enough. I would bet that you've heard this effective combination from an authority figure. Again, it's annoying that we must even consider changes like these. And you don't have to alter your normal tone of voice all the time, or ever for that matter. However, the unfortunate reality is that these cues, being unconscious and universal, are what they are, and they affect us all. Just as animals use posturing and various sounds to communicate with each other, we communicate far more with non-verbals and tone than most of us realize.

If it still irritates you to make these changes, then consider this: they may be after a certain reaction that you can deny them. Instead, give them something they don't expect or won't enjoy. If our voices are raised, if we get flustered or emotional, that may be part of what they want. Don't give it to them. Use crisp and clear speech, as though you were issuing commands. Try to avoid "filler" words such as "um", "like", or "you know" between sentences, as well as expressions such as "I guess" or "ok". Vocal cues of confidence are vitally important with someone who is being inappropriate or making you nervous. These last few suggestions are common in business books for women, as they help us sound more professional and composed overall.

Last but not least, many women and girls giggle when they are nervous. I know, because I was a giggler. This is not good. My guy friends told me that giggling is a huge "green light" for men. They don't realize that we are nervous or uncomfortable; instead, they interpret our giggling as a sign that we like whatever it is they are saying or doing. Bite your tongue if you need to—just don't giggle.

CHAPTER 7

FINDING YOUR INNER
FIGHTING SPIRIT

While you're practicing your new non-verbals and starting to appear more confident, you can also practice assertiveness skills. If the idea of standing up for yourself is too much, then you can begin with small steps in everyday situations.

To make this fun, you might want to choose a warrior name or image for this new facet of yourself. Search for someone who inspires you, a role model whose energy you can channel as you stretch beyond your comfort zone and find your voice. One woman told me that her warrior spirit was a ninja. Choose a legendary warrior, superhero/heroine, mythological god or goddess, historical figure, or contemporary influencer that resonates with you. Then, let them flow through you when you need a little courage, just as Boudicca did for me.

Old mindset: "I can't say anything" or, "I don't know what to do."
New mindset: "I can express myself confidently."

The first challenge is to stop saying, "I'm sorry" whenever somebody walks in front of or bumps into you—and for everything else. Women habitually apologize. Even when asking a question, women often apologize first. Stop it. It would be better for us if we eliminated this tendency, as it is submissive. In re-training myself, I used the expression "Oops!", instead. You can also say "Excuse me", depending on the circumstances, although in addition to trying to break the habit of the constant "Sorry", this is very much about realizing that we only need to apologize when we have done something wrong.

Pick up any business book for women and the author will probably make this point. My favorites are *How to Say It for Women*, by Phyllis Mindell, and *Nice Girls Don't Get the Corner Office*, by Lois Frankel. Notice these titles. We benefit when we speak up and get over the habit of being too nice.

Another way to practice confidence and assertiveness is to ask for clarification. In a fantastic little book called *The Four Agreements* by Don Miguel Ruiz, the Third Agreement is don't make assumptions. The problem with assumptions is that, after we make them, we accept them as fact and act accordingly. The solution is to seek clarification.

Instead of guessing or assuming, we ask questions. Confident people are comfortable saying things like, "Can you explain that?" or, "I'm not sure what you're getting at", because they understand that no one knows everything. It's fine to admit to gaps in our knowledge and to question misunderstandings or miscommunications, because we all have them. I have to do this with tech all the time—most eight-year-olds are better with technology than I am.

Find your voice. Practice saying what you need or would like to happen, starting with your friends and family, then working your way up to coworkers, authority figures, etc. Politely yet firmly express your preferences when asked. And, as you get better at this, express your preferences even when you haven't been asked.

In our attempts to be nice and get along, we women often bite our tongues and let others have their way. While reality dictates that we don't always get our way, this can be a good first step in the practice of speaking up. Be prepared for a "no", or to compromise, but don't let this stop you from speaking up again.

Try objecting when necessary. My favorite role model, Ms. Janis Ware, very politely but firmly uses phrases like, "That doesn't work for me", "This is unacceptable", and "This does not make me happy". Notice the absence of the word "sorry". Practicing these phrases during your regular daily activities will build confidence and assertiveness while you still maintain an air of politeness. Tone is everything, so work on keeping your voice low and calm.

Practice saying "No". Janis taught me that "No" is a complete sentence. You don't need to say more. If you feel like you must explain, then you can add, "That (day/time/whatever) doesn't work for me" or, "I can't help you with that." Or, "I already have too much on my plate". Don't feel that you need to make a long list of excuses. Keep it short and simple, then hold your position. You can smile and be sympathetic, but experiment with not giving in.

While this is technically about over-committing, the application works as it builds general self-esteem and confidence to establish your boundaries, which will benefit you in all areas of your life. If you are feeling guilty about saying "no", Janis has a mantra for that, too: "This is not my problem." While she mostly says this to herself, she has gently said it to others who were not taking a hint. You don't have to take on everyone's problems; you are not obligated to fix everything.

In uncomfortable situations with men or bullies, it's important to say "No" soon—and often, if necessary. Establish your boundary! If a guy politely asks me out, I'll say, "No, thanks." If he's not polite, pushes the issue, or makes an unacceptable request, then it's a firm "No" or one of the other responses we will cover shortly. In cases of repeated harassment, it's critical that we, at the very least, say "No". If we let it slide more than once, it will be perceived as a "green light": "Well, she didn't say no..." This has been used against us far too many times. Let's take that away from them, too, by learning to say "No".

Last but not least, during my time in the film industry, I had an amazing, well-known actor as a client. Her ability to face a difficult or uncomfortable situation head-on was extraordinary, especially since she was only in her twenties. She would say something like, "I have this challenging situation that I'm hoping you can help me navigate. What do you suggest we do about...?" This approach was assertive yet diplomatic and disarming, which was a powerful combination for dealing with situations she preferred to remedy, rather than burn a bridge.

Practice these strategies until they come naturally. As you do, you will begin to feel more confident and assertive, and retrain your brain at the same time.

CHAPTER 8

Resilience/Mental Toughness

It used to be that when people felt someone needed to be tougher, they would say the person needed "thicker skin", which meant they were going to pick on them more often to make them tougher. We now recognize this as just another form of bullying. Instead, let's think of "thicker skin" as resilience, a strengthened spirit, mental toughness, or a mindset where you realize, at your core, that you have value. Then, the words and actions of others won't be as hurtful.

This lesson is hammered into boys, who end up suppressing a whole different set of emotions than girls are conditioned to suppress. Yet, we can *choose* to become more resilient. It's a mean world out there, and there will invariably be things that will be upsetting, so what have you got to lose?

We tend to think that our mental and emotional characteristics are what they are, and that we are simply stuck being this way or that way for the rest of our lives. Nope. Remember that brain science says otherwise. We can choose better, more functional ideas or thoughts, and create better habits and behaviors through repetition and training.

The key word here is "training". There is no magical, quick fix. The closest I've seen to a quick fix is hypnosis, which I've used since my teens. But you still might need multiple sessions. Changing mindsets will take three-to-four weeks, at a minimum, because that's how long it takes to form a new habit. Deeply held beliefs may take months to change. Would an outcome of an easier life make this effort worth it?

Earlier, I mentioned Cognitive Behavioral Therapy (CBT), which holds that our thoughts control our emotions. By paying attention to and learning to control our thoughts, we can manage our emotions. But, since I do not hold a degree in psychology, I'm going to offer another option.

A few years ago, I got into the philosophy of Stoicism. During a visit to my psychiatrist, I mentioned making a daily practice of studying it. He told me that Albert Ellis, the psychologist who had come up with Rational Emotive Therapy (the first form of CBT), was inspired by the Stoics.

Stoicism is easy to access. You don't have to see a psychologist, although I still highly recommend mental health check-ups for, well, pretty much all of us. You can find plenty of information on Stoicism online, including videos on Youtube and the works of the original Stoics as well as contemporary authors. My current favorite is *The Daily Stoic* by Ryan Holiday, because he gives you a daily quote from a philosopher and then makes it easy to understand how to apply this timeless wisdom to your life.

Stoicism is meant to be studied daily, for a few minutes in the morning to get you off on the right foot, and then later, if needed, to get you back on track or to evaluate how you did at the end of the day. It focuses on the fact that so much of our lives is not under our control. We can't control external events or other people. The Stoics believed that letting our happiness and self-worth be affected by what we cannot control led to lots of unhappiness, anger, and disappointment. However, we can learn to take charge of how we interpret events as well as the words and actions of others.

We just—and I know this is a huge "just"—need to change our expectations. We tend to think we're entitled to things working out the way we hope or expect they "should"—maybe because we worked hard for a particular outcome, or maybe just because we wanted so much for things to be a certain way. And then, when they don't work out, we are disappointed or unhappy.

Stoicism gives us power over our thoughts and feelings. I know it sounds crazy, maybe even impossible, but this philosophy works. All it takes is practice, and the effort that you put into this will yield amazing results in all aspects of your life. Stoicism can help you become resilient. Practicing this philosophy can help you become immune to the cruelty of other people and the world. We can realize that what people say to us doesn't matter. We can choose to not react, to just ignore it. What matters is that we know who we are, that we love and respect ourselves.

When you get good at this, it is unbelievably liberating. Imagine not spending any more time worrying about what someone said, or what they might have meant, or if you might have done something wrong because this or that happened. Can you imagine having all that mental energy freed up for other things?

Again, I'm guessing you might be feeling that this is just too hard, if not impossible. I get it, because I remember feeling that way when I first encountered these ideas. But I found that by keeping my mind open, giving it a try, learning and applying the ideas, I was freed from the horrible thoughts that constantly ran through my mind. You can do this, too.

And we are not limited to Stoicism or Cognitive Behavioral Therapy. These concepts have appeared in the works of many philosophers, scholars, writers and poets throughout the ages. Dr. Viktor Frankl, in his book *Man's Search for Meaning,* details his practice of this while he was a prisoner in a concentration camp in WWII. He had lost everything and everyone, and yet realized he could still control his thoughts. The work he created from his experiences is called "Logos Therapy", from the Latin *logos,* or "word", although the larger meaning is "wisdom" or "the way".

In *The Four Agreements,* this concept is Agreement Number Two, which says to not take anything personally. Everything people say and do to us is about something going on with them. This is a variation of the adage "You cannot love or hate something about another person unless it's a reflection of something you love or hate about yourself".

Dr. Deepak Chopra discusses a similar idea in his book, *The Seven Spiritual Laws of Success,* in Law Number Four. It's the law about releasing attachment, in this case attachment to a specific outcome. Or, as I phrased it earlier, the idea that just because we want or worked for something, things will turn out a specific way. The Buddha said that desire is the cause of all human suffering, as in desire for a specific outcome. Same idea, different phrasing. The concept has been regenerated for millennia.

CHAPTER 9

Dealing with Violations of our Dignity and Boundaries

Have you ever had something happen and you basically froze, and then for the next hours/days/weeks you thought about what you should have said or done? Let's detour into the science on that for a minute—can you tell that I love science?

Most of us have probably heard of the "fight or flight" response to danger. Well, those aren't the only options. There is also freezing, which scientists call *tonic immobility*. It is an automatic, instinctive, and common response to trauma. A recent Swedish study of sexual assault victims found that 70% reported significant freezing and 48% reported extreme freezing during various stages of an assault—and it's not just women. Men also freeze in traumatic or life-threatening situations.

If you get nothing else from this book, please know that, if you freeze, it's still not your fault!

Everyone experiences fear. It has been said that the heroes among us respond despite their fears. The best way to get to a place where you can respond, even when you're afraid, is training. Repetition. Over and over, so you develop a reflexive response.

You might be thinking, *How am I going to get this training?* That's an excellent question. You could study a martial art. Or, believe it or not, you can do a lot by imagining. The use of creative visualization provides your brain with the practice you need. Although it works best when you use detailed visualizations, even a little is better than nothing—just slip it into some of your daydreams. Seriously. I know that I'm asking you to do some really weird daydreaming, but if you do it, it can help. When I began this part of training, I would recall specific incidents, then substitute a better response in my visualization instead of what really happened, which was usually freezing and not saying anything. Or, I'd be standing in line at the grocery store or post office, imagining what, *exactly*, I would do if someone grabbed me.

This technique is from a book called *Psycho-Cybernetics* by Maxwell Maltz, M.D., which was first published in 1960. It's a powerful book that has inspired the entire industry of motivational speakers. It's been used by professional and Olympic athletes and people from all walks of life to improve their performance in any number of situations. Maltz detailed how creative visualization and mental rehearsing can be effective tools to make changes in your life.

Now, let's go on to the next step.

New mindset: "I can stand up for myself when needed."

As we learn to stand up for ourselves, let's always go for a scaled response to boundary violations. This means that we will choose a response that is appropriate for the problem. So, verbal harassment gets a verbal response. Do not, I repeat, do *not* use a physical response to a verbal comment, unless the person is right on top of you or backing you into a corner. If you respond physically to a verbal comment, then you have committed assault. However, if they touch you, then a physical response is warranted and defensible. We don't touch them first, but when it comes to bullies, my daddy used to say, "If they start it, you can finish it."

CHAPTER 10

RESPONDING TO VERBAL HARASSMENT

We can get past freezing by taking a deep breath to focus, then using one of the simple responses you've chosen and practiced. Remember or imagine a few situations where you could use your phrases to defend yourself with a positive outcome. Try practicing with your friends or saying them in front of a mirror when you can. When you can't, then creative visualization counts as training, as it creates and reinforces new pathways in the brain, changing your mindset to one where you speak up for yourself.

First, you can always just ignore comments and refuse to engage. If you adopt a neutral, relaxed body stance and pretend that an offender is invisible, this can be effective. You don't have to acknowledge or answer harassment, bullying, or body-shaming. Ignoring can be a good option, especially if you can leave. Why? Sometimes, they are in it for the reaction. If you don't show one, it takes the fun out of it for them. Your disinterest shuts them down. But I'd only recommend doing that once. Repeat offenses must be addressed, or you will appear to be an easy target. If it's not the first time, or you can't leave, let's look at your options.

First, you can ask a question. In general, try to keep your posture relaxed and your voice calm. "What did you say?" "What do you mean?"

"Why would you say something like that?"

"What would your mama think about what you just said?"

The above responses, delivered in a calm, maybe even slightly humorous way, would give the guy a chance to back off and save face. This is a good first choice if you are alone with the person or again, if they are your boss, a superior, an authority figure, or someone with whom you must interact regularly.

Another option is active listening, where you paraphrase and repeat back to them what they said. For example, "Just to be clear, you're asking me to...?" Let them hear how their own words sound. Add a look of genuine confusion on your face to help throw them off their game.

If you're feeling more confident, you could also make a firm statement. Again, shoot for a neutral, relaxed posture and a low, neutral tone of voice. It's also fine to just stare at them for a couple of seconds as you choose your reply. A short, uncomfortable silence can be a good start.

"Stop it."

"Enough."

"I'm not interested."

"That is inappropriate."

"Dude, not cool."

"I'm taken/unavailable." (Even if you aren't).

Ok, I'm officially giving you permission to lie, if needed, as this was easier for me when I first started learning to resist. While it would be nice if we didn't have to claim having a boyfriend or husband to get men to leave us alone, the reality is that it can be an easy way out. This is because, while men may not respect *our* right to choose whether we wish to engage with them, some will respect another man's "property". It annoys me to write that, but this is the world we live in. So, if that seems like the easiest, safest way to do it, then go for it.

On the other hand, there are also plenty of men who don't care either way. I've had men who knew I was married hit on me anyway. The night after taking my workshop, a friend—let's call her "Cassandra"—was staying the night at the house of some friends. She awoke to a guy trying to fondle her breasts—someone who was friends with her boyfriend.

She slapped him across the face and he slunk away into another room, giving her the opportunity to leave. The next day, she received an apology letter from the guy, and she told me that she felt good knowing her actions had stopped him.

Unsurprisingly, Cassandra's story got more complicated when the guy took a different approach a few days later, blaming his actions on her for hanging out with a group of mostly guys, drinking and discussing sex. But she wasn't having it. She had realized that it wasn't her fault, and she held strong and got through the backlash. And, she still had the letter in case things escalated.

It sounds simple, but it is always harder to do in the moment, right? Just remember, the trick is to have some responses ready to go. Practice/ imagine using a couple of questions or phrases that seem right for you, so that you create a mindset where you can speak up for yourself. Personally, I often pretend to be really confused or make it into a joke to throw back at them, keeping things light while still letting them know their "crap wont' fly". Feel free to come up with others, although I highly recommend, in the spirit of not escalating, that you avoid snarky or insulting comebacks. Once upon a time, if it was a guy in your social circle or at work or school, we could take that approach—but I don't recommend that now. It's safer to de-escalate.

What if you don't manage to respond in the moment? Don't sweat it—it takes practice. If it's someone whom you work with or is still around, you can always approach them and express yourself in the next few minutes or hours, or even the next day. Just try not to let it go much longer than that. If you need to, give yourself a minute to think about what you want to say. Then go practice your confidence non-verbals and your assertiveness skills. Make sure to use a calm, low tone with your strong posture and confident speech, and keep it short and direct. For example: "I was surprised by what you said a few (minutes/hours) ago, but it is unacceptable and inappropriate, and I will not put up with that kind of talk." You can do this, even if you have to channel your warrior role model to assist you.

There are a several possible outcomes for what happens next. Often, the guy will stop, leave, or even apologize. However, some will protest you protesting, as in "How dare you call me on my bad behavior?" They might say they were joking and accuse you of lacking a sense of humor. To them, I say, "Not funny". While you're building your confidence, you might prefer to use, "I don't get it". They might say you imagined it or call you crazy. This is gaslighting. My response is, "My hearing is fine".

And, of course, they can resort to calling us names: "crazy", "bitch", "slut", "skank", "ball-buster", "cold", "no fun", etc. Because what happens when they call us names? We often stop protesting. At our core, most of us still need to think of ourselves as "nice". Once again, I got over that, and you can, too. You can still be nice 99% of the time, but **you don't have to be nice to someone who is harassing you.**

Learning to not be bothered by name calling is tough at first. It begins with understanding that the fear of being perceived as "not nice" comes from social messaging. This is about how others want us to behave. It's part of how men (and other women) have gotten women to submit for centuries. Just the thought of being anything but nice can make many women feel guilty. They call us a name, and we shut up. Many women have told me that name-calling feels like a slap in the face or a punch in the gut. Words do have power, and they use them against us. Try to see name-calling for the manipulation it is.

Recently, a friend told me a story of a guy she was occasionally walking dogs with in her neighborhood. Somewhere along the line, this married guy got it into his head that they were going to be hanging out and having drinks. When this didn't happen because of her work and personal obligations, he sent a series of late-night texts that were creepy and angry. Most striking to me was when he called her "selfish" and suggested that she only put on a polite, engaging front. He felt entitled to her time, and when she didn't give it, he chastened her. She really had just thought they were walking dogs together, and that he understood she was busy since she had told him as much.

My new mindset is, "They can call me whatever they want, as long as they stay away from me". For the record, when someone calls me a name, if I respond, it will be with something like, "So, you're reduced to name-calling now?" or "Why are you calling me a name?".

In general, most women could be much more assertive and still be far from bitchy. When you're called this, or worse, it's because you resisted, in which case, good for you! See it for what it is: a pathetic attempt to shame you into taking someone's crap.

Here's the good news: most of the time, this step works—even if he calls you a name. You've shown him you're not an easy target and are going to stand up for yourself. But, if this doesn't stop it, then we might need to enforce our boundaries more confidently and forcefully—*loudly*, if needed.

"STOP!"

"BACK OFF!"

"DON'T TALK TO ME THAT WAY!"

"LEAVE ME ALONE!"

"I'VE TOLD YOU I'M NOT INTERESTED!"

"ENOUGH!"

"DUDE! I'VE TOLD YOU THIS IS NOT COOL!"

If it's at school or work and you see this person often, make a note of it with date, time, and a description of the events including your response, and email it to someone or file it away. If it happens again, record the incident, what they said or did, with your response, which might include a reminder that this is the second time they've said something inappropriate, and email or file it again. On the third time, record everything again and then take your records to someone in a position of authority. It's important to document, document, document. Keep a written account and make a paper trail!

So, these are the easier situations. Next, what do we do when they touch or grab us?

CHAPTER 11

DEALING WITH
UNWANTED TOUCHING

These are the incidents where it's so common to freeze. But, just like any other skill, you can train yourself to respond. If you practice enough (even just mentally), it can become a reflex.

First, take a deep breath and focus. Depending on the context and other variables, you could, in a very commanding tone, say something like, "That's not appropriate", while you gently (or not) brush their hands off you. You may want or need to take this approach if it's someone with whom you want or need to preserve a relationship.

If you'd rather not get physical, you can use a strong and loud voice as you step away from them:

"DON'T TOUCH ME!"

"GET YOUR HANDS OFF ME!"

And it's completely ok if you don't want to physically fight back. If you're in public, get loud to attract the attention of other people. In many places these days, it will be caught on video, which is to our advantage. *Use this advantage.*

Or, if you want, your loud, verbal response could be accompanied by a physical move. When you choose this, get into it. Call on your fighting spirit. Use some force, putting your body weight behind whatever you do. Striking is not about hitting or kicking—it's about directing your energy through your body (via your elbow, knee, whatever) to a point a few inches *beyond* your target. We don't aim at the target, as that limits the force of the strike. Instead, we aim *behind* the target, to deliver more energy.

Options:

1. Slap their hand away from you. The sound of a slap is often more of a jolt than the slap itself.
2. Use the knife edge of your hand (from the base of the pinkie finger to the wrist) to dislodge their hand(s).
3. If they have a tighter grip on you, grab their pinkie finger and quickly jerk it backward and down. Hard. And, step behind or away from them while you do this, in case their other hand comes at you.
4. Elbow them if they are behind you and close. Aim for their solar plexus, up under their chin, or at their jaw or nose. I elbowed a coworker once, followed by an "Oops! You surprised me when you snuck up and grabbed me! Don't do that again because I have these weird reflexes", all with an innocent and surprised look on my face. He never touched me again.
5. Knee them when they are in front of you. Grab them by their clothes and pull them into your knee.
6. Donkey kick if they are behind you (especially if you have something to hold on to). This would have been ideal for my friend who was bent over when she got her buttocks smacked. She had something to grab and the kick would have been powerful.
7. Stomp on their instep. Don't step—STOMP! Put your weight behind it.

There's a lot of room for variation in the severity of your response in any given situation. How do you choose? How do you know what to do? There are many factors to consider, so you may want to do that weird day-dreaming/imagining thing I mentioned earlier, to help you decide how you might respond to different situations.

Do you remember an incident that you or someone you know had in the past? Imagine a different ending to that event. Has someone been bothering you, like my friend who had a coworker who grabbed every-one? Imagine how you might react next time. Cultivate a "What if?" mindset. I do this often when I'm standing in line for something. Instead of checking social media, I imagine what I would do "if". A little bit of mental rehearsing can feel really empowering and help train your brain to respond.

When choosing a response, only you can evaluate all the factors. For instance, is the person an acquaintance or a stranger? Boss or coworker? Teacher or another student? Are you in a public place, or are you isolated? Where is their body in relation to yours? Each of these will play a role in how you respond.

You must do what feels right for you in the moment. Listen to your gut. We've been taught to ignore our instincts and give everyone else the benefit of the doubt. If you honor your instincts, they'll get better. In his book, *The Gift of Fear,* Gavin de Becker emphasizes learning to value your instincts and bodily responses—like your stomach turning or the hair standing up on the back of your neck. These are signs of impending dan-ger, so you might want to run or call on your inner fighting spirit if you can't run away.

Many people are going to respond physically only as a last resort, and that's understandable. It means you're civilized and not a violent person, and that's a good thing *most* of the time. I'm a big fan of de-escalation in general, but I have no patience with unwanted touching. I didn't teach slapping the face, but that's what Cassandra did naturally, as her attacker had her at a major disadvantage. It was an excellent choice. Weeks after the incident, she told me she felt confident and that she was no longer going to be manipulated into feeling bad or guilty when it wasn't her fault. This was a big win!

If you're scared, if you feel the hair on the back of your neck standing up, or you've had another experience that makes you want to fight back, then channel your inner fighting spirit and release your warrior self! Or, just yell at them. There is no need to feel obligated to be nice to someone who isn't being nice to you. I know I've said that before, but it's a critical point. **You are worth fighting for, even if you must do it yourself. You are worthy of respect and dignity, and your body isn't public property. But again, if you freeze, please remember that this is a normal response, and do not blame yourself.** Direct any bad feelings toward *them*—where they belong.

And this is important: they are not expecting us to fight back. This is to our advantage, as it gives us the element of surprise. Between this and the otherwise lamentable presence of cameras everywhere, we have a couple of things in our favor.

CHAPTER 12

RELEASING YOUR WARRIOR SELF

Disclaimer: I don't have a black belt. I'm not a trained or certified self- defense instructor. At first, I thought this might be a problem. But when I started surveying people, friends, and acquaintances with lots of training, and those with none, it turned out that my non-expert status was fine. In fact, I was told it's less intimidating and the women who participate can more easily relate.

Because I was truly over it all, I *did* take eighteen months of *Hagganah*, a vicious Israeli military self-defense system. Between that and the help of some guy friends who ranged from Special Forces to black belts in a variety of martial arts, I've chosen the moves that are safest and most effective for women and girls who have little to no training.

Basic self-defense skills:

1. **Awareness**—Prevention is key. Many of you know this, but I'm going to review it anyway. Be aware of your surroundings and who is there, especially who is watching you. Harassment and assault, like robbery and theft, are crimes of opportunity. We want to reduce opportunity. Perps are looking to catch you off-guard, with your thoughts elsewhere. Speaking of which, you

cannot be aware of your surroundings if you're texting, talking on the phone, or exercising outside with headphones.

2. **Avoidance**—Think ahead about parking, the path you have to walk outside or inside, and be aware of potential exits in any building. Practice a "What if?" mindset. Most of us do this automatically, as we have been conditioned to be careful. A social researcher named Jackson Katz once took an audience survey. First, he asked the men what they did on a daily basis to avoid sexual assault. The response was that they didn't think about it. Then, he asked the women: their list was past thirty things when Katz stopped writing them down.

Most of us are already thinking about these things. Unfortunately, we cannot afford to let down our guard. It's horrifically unfair, but life isn't fair, and we must work with the world as it is and not as we wish it to be.

More important tips include:

Use the buddy system. Please go to parties or clubs with at least one friend and do not, under any circumstances, get separated from them. No matter how cute or hot some guy is, don't go off with him or allow your friend to do so either. If he is worth it, he will be fine with a date at another time. I'm not going to list the well-known cases where ignoring this rule resulted in tragedy. And, even so, **it STILL wasn't their fault.** I keep repeating that, because it's so important that we get past the self-blame and shame.

Most of us know not to take drinks from people and to not leave your drink unattended. The few times I went to house or frat parties, I'd either switch the drinks they gave me with a distracted guy, or pretend to drink it, then dump it out somewhere.

Please be careful with alcohol or other drugs. Once you lose control, you are at someone's mercy, and I've met multiple women who were raped under those circumstances. **Again, it wasn't their fault. The blame always belongs to the one committing the assault.**

Here's my favorite hack: if you must go to a house party, or you intend to party hard anywhere, wear jeans or pants with a zipper. Then, take a small safety pin and put it under the zipper tab at the top. *TaDa!* Your pants are now really hard to take off. Just make sure you leave a little early for the bathroom, because you might need a minute longer. I learned that trick as a teenager, and it saved me a few times from unwanted undressing. This was why the guys in the "group grope" couldn't unzip my jeans when they tried.

So, what if none of that helped? You're cornered, outnumbered, or otherwise disadvantaged. Now what?

3. Get loud and push back hard. "BACK OFF!!"

Hurt them quickly. Reach deep down inside for some anger, tap into your inner fighting spirit, and release your inner warrior! Expert fighters will try to avoid the fight if possible, and so should we. But when we must fight, we need to strike quickly and effectively to give us time to get away. We do not want to be trading punches and kicks, as we will surely lose— we must be fast and vicious.

Speaking of punches, even trained fighters will break their fingers when punching, so I can't recommend using your fists to strike. There are several good options though, which are surprisingly instinctual moves (remember the "group grope"?). And again, striking isn't about punching or kicking—it's about focusing your body weight strategically toward a point beyond your actual target.

Best Targets and Moves:

1. **Eyes**—Use your fingers (tight together), your thumb, a knuckle, keys, or anything you can get. Poke hard!

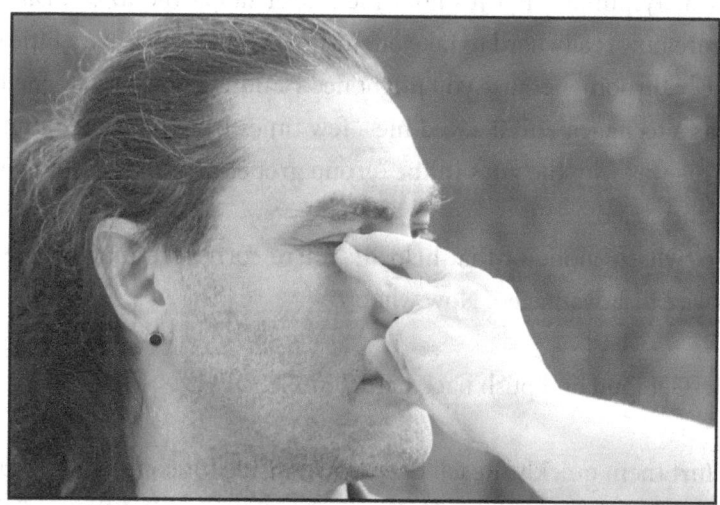

2. **Nose**—Use the heel of your hand and come from under the nose, driving upward.

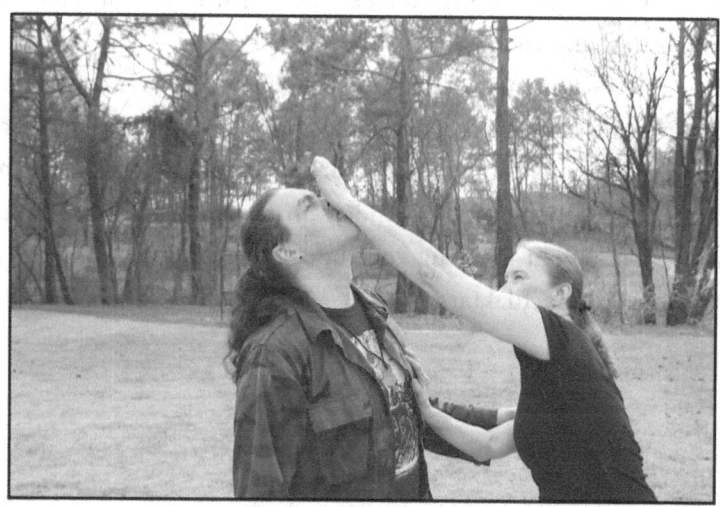

3. **Jaw**- Use elbow when they are behind you

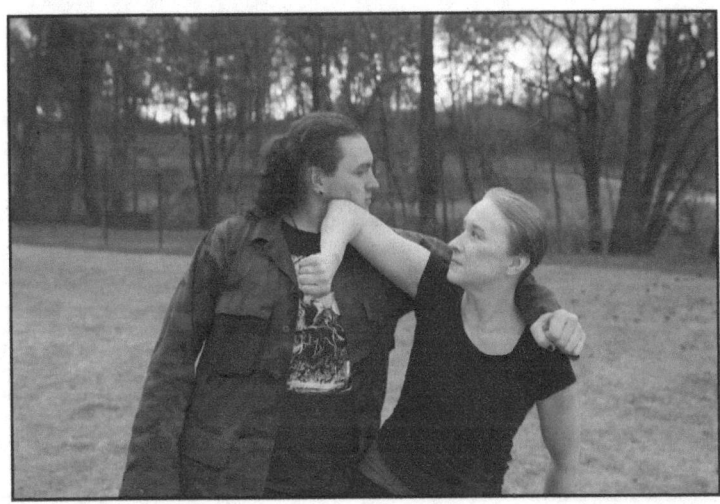

4. **Throat**—Use the "V" between thumb and first finger if they are in front of you, or your elbow if they are behind you. Aim behind the Adam's Apple.

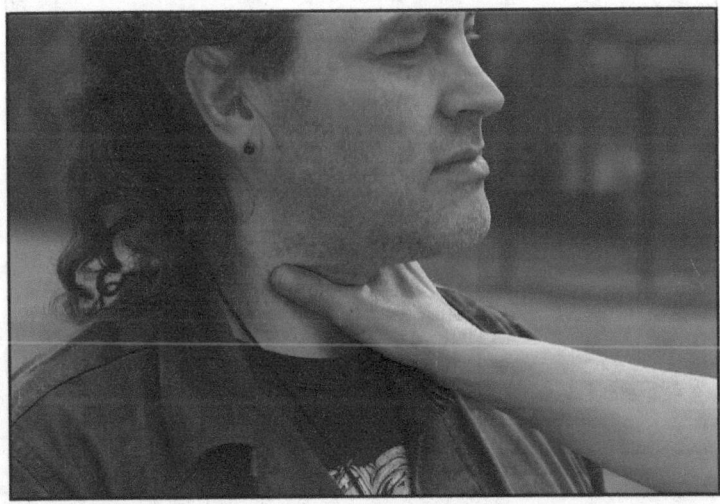

5. **Solar plexus**—Use elbow if they are behind you

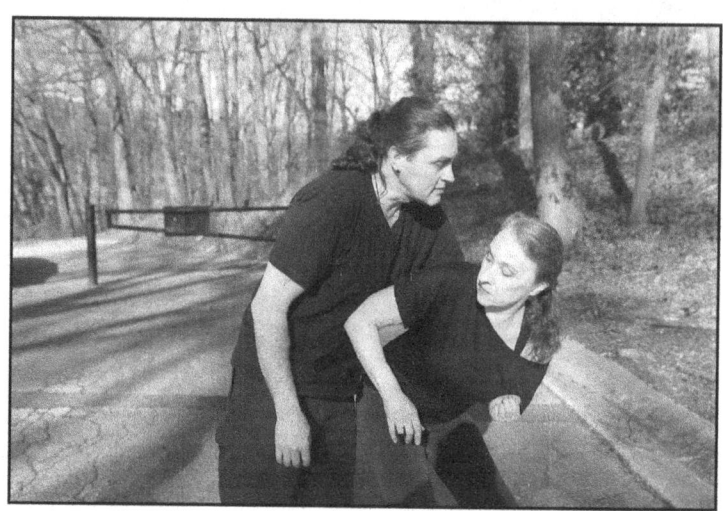

6. **Groin**—Grab their shirt/coat or arms and pull them into your knee.

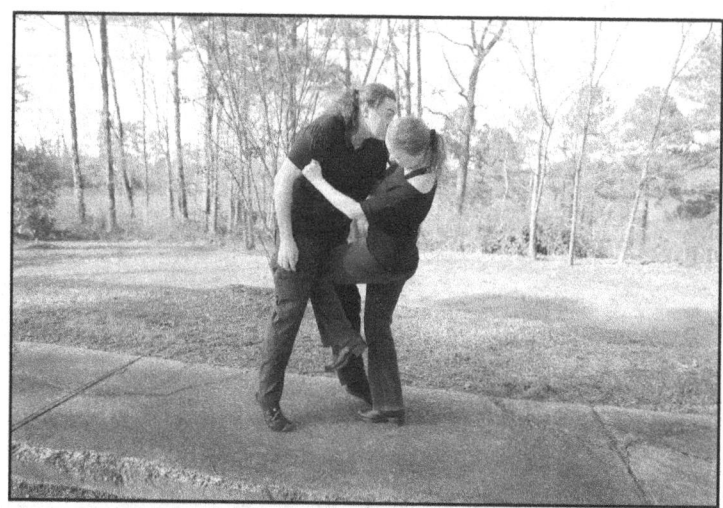

7. **Knees**—My favorite target. Kick hard from most angles and they won't be chasing you.

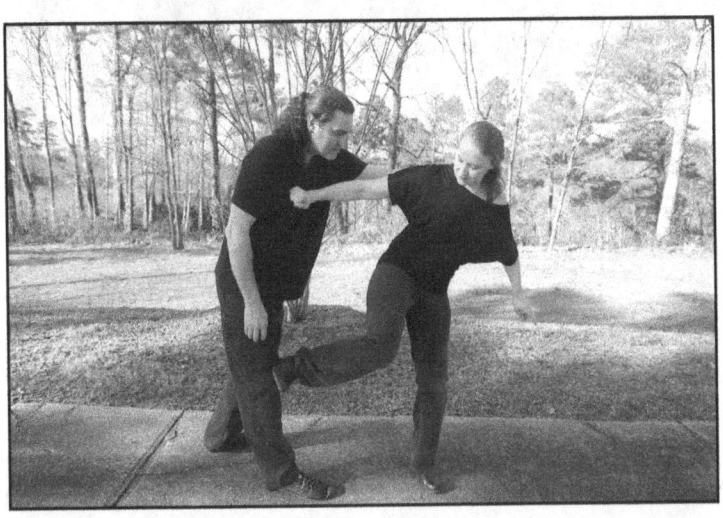

8. **Feet**—Stomp on their instep, on the top of the foot.

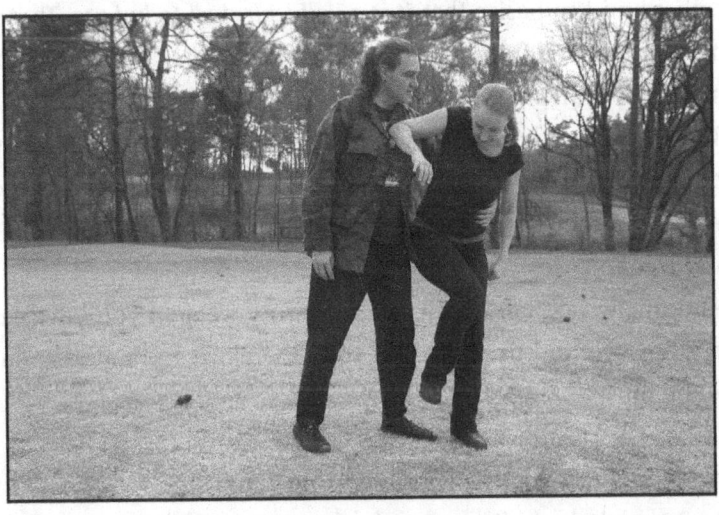

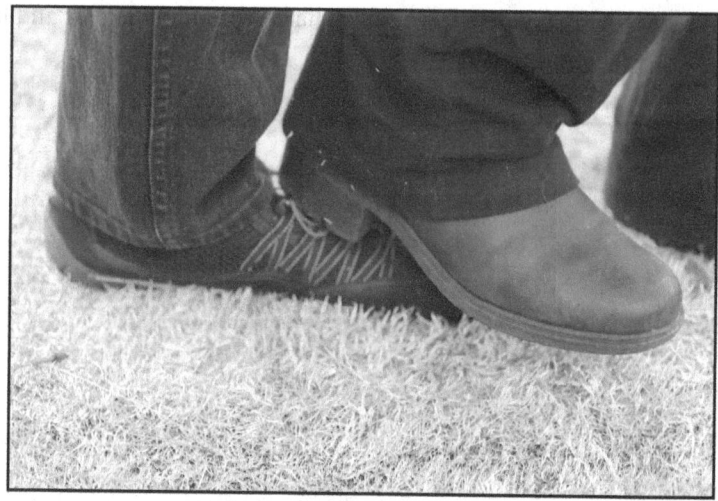

Note: While it is often in our best interest to resist/fight back, there are circumstances where surrendering may save us from more violence or even save our lives. If we must make this horrible choice, then we need to remember and emphasize that *it is a valid survival technique.* Therefore, we must be liberated from the lie that this puts any blame or shame on us or diminishes us in any way.

The exception to this rule is if they are trying to get you into a vehicle to take you somewhere else. Experts agree: do not go to the second scene—even if they have a weapon. It's statistically better to fight back at the first scene.

And finally, let's talk about weapons: **Any weapon you have can be taken from you and used against you**. Therefore, for any weapon you carry, you must:

1. Train. Practice deploying and using it.
2. Be psychologically prepared to use it.
3. Use it immediately after deploying. No brandishing it as a threat, because that's how it gets taken away.

For a few years, I had a business that involved travel. After the third law enforcement official told me that I should have a gun, I decided to purchase one—especially since my first stalker was still out there. Plus, there was a serial rapist in Florida at that time, prowling Interstate 95, which I often took for work (The rapist turned out to be a state trooper, so having a weapon wouldn't have helped in that situation).

Anyway, I bought a gun. I took the required weekend class to get my concealed-carry permit. Then, I took lots of private lessons to learn how to draw the gun from a specialized purse. I spent many hours practicing at the range, and I carried that gun for twenty years.

And then, when I began feeling more confident, I started leaving my gun at home. Not too long after that, lots and lots more people started carrying. Then the mass shootings started and became more and more frequent. In a couple of incidents, good guys who were trying to help got shot, sometimes by police who arrived at the scene and didn't know that the guy with the gun was trying to help—because you're not supposed to try to help. My instructors had made it crystal clear that we were still supposed to run away, not run toward the shooting with our guns drawn like an action hero wannabe.

And so, I stopped carrying. Now I have a personal alarm that makes a loud noise when the pin is pulled. Please get something like this for yourself.

CONCLUSION

It is my hope that this information will help speed your transformation to a confident and assertive woman, in touch with her inner fighting spirit and warrior self. This confidence will help you in all areas and aspects of your life, and you'll be more prepared to deal with any incidents that may arise. If you read at least a few of the recommended books, use repetition techniques to change your mindsets, practice the nonverbal confidence behaviors, the assertiveness exercises, the verbal responses and physical moves, your life will be so much easier.

Most incidents can be managed verbally, with an assertive yet calm demeanor and a relaxed tone of voice. In situations of physical contact, you now have a good start on knowing what to say and do, however the basic self-defense moves I've covered here are just that: a starting point. Therefore, I'll finish by encouraging you to take a self-defense course. Even better, if you've ever thought of taking up a martial art, go for it!

If more of us stand up for ourselves, I believe we can start a ripple effect that will help other women and girls, too. If creeps meet more resistance, they might think twice before trying again.

As Maya Angelou said, "Each time a woman stands up for herself, without knowing it, possibly, without claiming it, she stands up FOR ALL WOMEN".

Recommended Reading

Love Yourself Like Your Life Depends on It by Kamal Ravikant

The Power of Now by Eckhart Tolle

The Daily Stoic by Ryan Holiday

The Four Agreements by Don Miguel Ruiz

Psycho-Cybernetics by Maxwell Maltz

How to Say It for Women, by Phyllis Mindell

Nice Girls Don't Get the Corner Office, by Lois Frankel

The Gift of Fear by Gavin de Becker

Check out my Instagram and YouTube channel, *Dr. Nora Fahlberg,* for related videos and information.

www.ingramcontent.com/pod-product-compliance
Lightning Source LLC
Chambersburg PA
CBHW011100280526
45785CB00008B/3050